Stoic Yoga

A Union of Mind and Body for Inner Strength

Table of Contents

Chapter 1. Introduction

In this Special Report, we delve into the enriching world of "Stoic Yoga: A Union of Mind and Body for Inner Strength". This isn't just your typical yoga exploration; we're bridging the power of ancient philosophy and physical discipline to forge an inner fortitude like none other! Here, you'll lay the groundwork for a lifestyle that embraces equilibrium, resilience, and tranquility even amid the tides of chaos. This is not a realm of esoteric theories; it's a practical, hands-on guide to boost your everyday life experience. Dive into this exciting fusion of Stoic wisdom and yogic practices to inspire your journey towards spiritual strength and mental balance. Purchase this report today and begin a transformative journey that will leave you rooting for more!

Chapter 2. Foundations of Stoic Yoga

To understand Stoic Yoga, we must first understand its two major components: Stoicism and Yoga, independently, before we can truly appreciate their union. This will help us to better conceptualize the potent blend of philosophy and physical practice that we aim to achieve.

2.1. Stoicism

Stoicism is said to have been introduced by Zeno of Citium around 300 BC, during the Hellenistic period in ancient Greece. The fundamental principle of Stoicism lies in distinguishing what we control from what we do not control.

In life, we often intermix the things we cannot change with those we can. For Stoics, the world within us - our feelings, thoughts, and volitions - lies in our control, whereas the world outside - other people, events, or the weather - is not within our domain. This inherent understanding promotes resilience, as it inspires peace despite external circumstances.

2.2. Yoga

On the other hand, Yoga, originating from ancient India, is a well-developed system for physical, mental, and spiritual well-being. Rooted in a rich spiritual tradition, Yoga aims to help practitioners attain inner peace by integrating the body, mind, and spirit. Its core components include ethical and moral guidelines, posture and physical exercises (asanas), breath control (pranayama), and meditation.

Now that we have grasped the core tenets of Stoicism and Yoga, we can start examining their fusion.

2.3. The Merger of Stoicism and Yoga

Stoicism teaches us to establish emotional equilibrium through the understanding of our control boundaries, while Yoga helps us to connect our mind, body, and spirit. When merged together, a holistic practice begins to form - a practice known as Stoic Yoga.

Stoic Yoga combines the mental toughness and emotional resilience of Stoicism with the physical discipline and awareness from Yoga. The combination of these two practices creates a potent tool for personal growth and inner peace, by making you both physically vital and mentally resilient.

2.4. Practice of Stoic Yoga

Like any practice, Stoic Yoga necessitates consistent dedication, an open mind, and a willing spirit. This session begins with stoic meditation to prime the mind, followed by yoga asanas for the body, and eventually, a tranquility meditation for a full embodiment of Stoic peace.

The stoic meditation is a contemplative exercise, focusing on discerning what we can and cannot control. This phase helps to prevent the mishap of getting caught up in situations beyond our control.

Subsequent is the yoga asanas stage. Every pose helps in tuning in to your body, and appreciating its strength and fragility. Through physical practice, we train our bodies and deepen the connection with our minds.

Ultimately, we close with a tranquility meditation. This session is aimed at engaging our mental and emotional faculties to promote a sense of calm and composure, in accordance with the Stoic ideal of tranquility.

By merging Stoicism and Yoga, we leverage the philosophical wisdom of the Greeks and the spiritual practices of the ancient Indians. Stoic Yoga offers a unique way to foster physical wellness, emotional resilience, and mental clarity. It is a holistic form of practice aimed at enhancing total human experience - a sturdy bridge between the mind and body.

2.5. Embodying Stoic Yoga in Daily Life

Stoic Yoga isn't just a one-time mediation or physical exercise - it is a transformative lifestyle. It's quietening the mind amid a storm, conducting yourself ethically, respecting your physical body, accepting change as part of life, and continuously striving for inner peace.

Remember, Stoic Yoga is a practice and not an end in itself. It's normal to falter and struggle in the initial stages or even later. That's part of the process. Be patient and extend understanding towards yourself, as you would do to anyone learning a new skill. Demonstrating a stoic attitude towards your progress in this journey is an achievement in itself.

In conclusion, Stoic Yoga envisages a life where we operate at our finest, not perturbed by external stimuli, dwelling peacefully within the realms of our control. It's about harnessing the power we hold over our thoughts, our mind and our bodies to live a balanced, resilient and calm life, regardless of circumstances. This form of mindful living is an ode to the ancient wisdom of Stoicism and Yoga, providing a pathway to inner strength this hectic 21st century deeply needs.

Chapter 3. Basics of Stoicism: History and Principles

In understanding the basics of Stoicism, it all begins with its origination, which dates back to around 300 BC in Athens, Greece. Stoicism, developed by Zeno of Citium, is a philosophy that emphasizes emotional resilience and personal virtue as paths to a good life. While Zeno established the teachings, it's also valuable to highlight a few essential contributors who expounded upon Stoic philosophy later. They are Epictetus (former slave and Stoic teacher), Seneca (a statesman, and advisor to Nero), and Marcus Aurelius (a Roman Emperor).

3.1. Stoicism: Imparted by the Ancients

Zeno, the pioneer of Stoicism, originally taught under a Stoa Poikile (painted porch), hence the name 'Stoicism'. Inspired by the teachings of Socrates and the Cynics, Zeno preached the importance of the harmonious life, which he believed could be obtained by aligning one's desires with nature's way. This deviated from the then prevalent pursuit of hedonistic pleasures and external achievements.

Epictetus, a prominent Stoic philosopher, was a powerful advocate of mental fortitude. Born a slave, he triumphed over his crude beginnings to become an esteemed philosopher. Epictetus proposed that we have no control over external events but can control our attitudes towards them. His teachings are beautifully summarized in his Enchiridion (Handbook), highlighting that freedom from suffering is achieved by distinguishing what is within our control from what isn't.

Seneca, the advisor to the infamous Nero, offered Stoic wisdom through his various letters and essays. His work highlighted the transient nature of life and the importance of living in accordance with nature. His writings are characterized by a deeply calming pragmatism, underscoring the need for rationality in the face of adversity.

Marcus Aurelius, the Roman emperor and Stoic philosopher, is best known for his 'Meditations.' His written work, never intended for publication, offers profound insight into the Stoic practice, often emphasizing duty, acceptance, and the transient nature of human existence.

3.2. Unraveling the Stoic Philosophy

Stoics teach that by developing a strong rapport with our minds and focusing on what is within our control, we can maintain tranquility and joy regardless of life's trials and tribulations. This philosophy boils down to four principal virtues: wisdom, courage, justice, and temperance.

Wisdom, to the Stoics, is the foundation of all virtues. It involves understanding the world, recognizing what is essential, and dealing with complexity logically and calmly. It's applied rationality in face of the world's intricate reality.

Courage is not only about physical bravery but consists of mental and emotional strength too. It's the nerve to stand in defence of wisdom and justice and manifests as the resilience to bear pain and adversity with fortitude.

Justice, from a Stoic perspective, involves fairness, generosity, and concern for the common welfare. It's the understanding that we are inseparably connected and must treat each other with dignity and respect.

Finally, temperance is about exercising self-control and moderation in all things. Mindful use of resources and balance in behavior are its key aspects.

3.3. Stoic Principles in Action

Stoicism involves a few basic principles that help in dealing with life's ups and downs. The first principle is to distinguish between what is within our control and what isn't. This understanding forms the basis for emotional resilience, as it allows us to accept what we can't change, thus freeing us to focus on what we can influence.

The second principle is to align our desires with nature—being satisfied with what is available to us naturally rather than pursuing unrelenting ambition and desire. In simpler terms, it means accepting and being content with the way things are instead of how we wish them to be.

The third principle is to see things for what they are. By removing our preconceived notions and biases, we can perceive the world more accurately and respond effectively. It involves stripping away the labels we apply to things and people, seeing them as they truly exist, in their purest forms.

Adopting the approach of Stoic indifference, the fourth principle, allows a person to remain unaffected by externals, be they good or bad. It doesn't mean to feel indifference but to comprehend that these externals do not define one's core essence.

The final principle is to live in accordance with nature, embracing life as it happens, with all its unpredictabilities and imperfections. This principle encourages us to adapt and survive, just as nature does, in the face of constant change.

Understanding and applying these Stoic principles is a transformative journey, a consistent practice that slowly seeps into one's thought patterns and behaviors, influencing daily life choices.

The beauty of Stoicism lies in its practicality and universal applicability, offering potent strategies for cultivating resilience, tranquillity, and personal strength.

As we move forward, we'll explore the enchanting world of yoga and examine the synergies between the physical discipline of yoga and the psychological strengthening of Stoicism. Together, they can create an unshakable inner strength—a fortified fortress of the mind and body, ready to endure the chaos of the world while still maintaining grace and tranquillity.

Chapter 4. Essential Yoga Practices: A Primer

At the intersection of Stoicism, a philosophy centered on emotional resilience and composure, and yoga, a holistic practice encompassing physical postures, breathing exercises, and meditation, lies a profound pathway to personal strength and inner tranquility. Together, these disciplines shine a light on the journey towards an enduring state of mind-body equilibrium.

4.1. The Fundamental Elements of Yoga

Understanding the core tenets of yoga is pivotal to grasp the intertwining with Stoicism and fully relishing their combined effect. Yoga is not merely a series of physical exercises; it incorporates a more profound sense of holistic wellness, which includes physical, mental, and spiritual elements.

4.1.1. Asanas - The Physical Postures

Asanas are the physical aspect of yoga, and they serve to enhance the body's flexibility, stamina, and strength. Far from being just a physical activity, asanas play a crucial role in the mind's alignment with the body. Every pose acts as a conduit for improved energy flow and a heightened sense of awareness.

Here lies a list of essential asanas that form the foundation for any yoga practice:

- *Tadasana (Mountain Pose)*: As the foundation of all standing poses, Tadasana aids in improving posture, balance, and calm focus.

- *Adho Mukha Svanasana (Downward-Facing Dog)*: This pose rejuvenates the body, stretching the shoulders, hamstrings, calves, arches, and hands, while calming the mind and improving digestion.

- *Balasana (Child's Pose)*: Balasana offers a unique sense of calmness and stability, providing physical, mental, and emotional relief.

- *Vrikshasana (Tree Pose)*: Vrikshasana is a balancing pose that hones concentration and strengthens the legs and back.

4.1.2. Pranayama - The Breathing Techniques

Pranayama involves the regulation of breath and serves to harness the life energy within us. The controlled practice of breathing ties in with the Stoic teaching of control and composure, enabling steadiness during grievous situations. Here are some common Pranayama techniques:

- *Anulom Vilom (Alternate Nostril Breathing)*: This involves inhaling and exhaling alternately through the nostrils, balancing the mind and enhancing concentration.

- *Kapalabhati (Skull Shining Breath)*: This technique is a rejuvenating practice that amplifies the body's energy and revitalizes the mind.

- *Ujjayi Pranayama (Victorious Breath)*: Known for its soft, whisper-like sound, Ujjayi Pranayama fosters an extended breath, promotes clear and focused mind, and provides a soothing and calming effect.

4.1.3. Dhyana - Meditation

Meditation, or Dhyana, stands as the bridge between the external and the internal, the physical and the metaphysical. It represents the journey from the self to the self, a discovery of our existence and potential to endure life's challenges. Meditation techniques that one could start with include:

- *Mindfulness Meditation*: Focusing on your breath without any attempt to control it. This heightens awareness and brings tranquility.

- *Loving-Kindness Meditation*: Directing well wishes and love towards yourself and those around you, urging an environment of kindness.

- *Candle Gazing Mediation or Trataka*: Focus remains on a single point - a candle flame - improving concentration power and cultivating mental resilience.

4.2. Complementing Yoga Practices with Stoic Philosophy

With a fundamental understanding of asanas, pranayama, and dhyana, we can look towards integrating the wisdom of Stoicism with these yogic practices. Stoicism, which emphasizes mental fortitude, teaches us the necessity of accepting what we cannot change, leading to a calm acceptance that greatly complements the tranquility sought through yoga.

From the physical resilience developed through asanas, the composed breath control of pranayama, to the mental clarity cultivated in meditation, every aspect of yoga converges seamlessly with Stoic teachings. Regular practice can lead to great heights in endurance, both in mind and body, establishing the inner strength to remain unaffected by external adversities.

4.3. Yoga Routine Infused with Stoic Wisdom

Define a daily yoga routine with stoic wisdom guiding the course. Here is an example:

1. Start with Tadasana (Mountain Pose), grounding yourself to the earth, and reflect upon the stoic principle of accepting the reality as it is.

2. Flow into Adho Mukha Svanasana (Downward-Facing Dog), channeling the stoic idea of emotional resilience to overcome physical discomfort.

3. Rest into Balasana (Child's Pose), focusing on controlling one's reactions, mirroring the stoic teaching of discipline.

4. End your asanas with Vrikshasana (Tree Pose), channeling stoic concentration to maintain balance and stability.

5. Transition into pranayama with Anulom Vilom, focusing on the dichotomy of control that Stoicism emphasizes.

6. Continue with Kapalabhati, invigorating your body and reflecting on the stoic principle of understanding and embracing life's transient nature.

7. Shift into Ujjayi pranayama, the Victorious Breath, symbolizing the mastery over adversities, a core stoic teaching.

8. Conclude your practice with Mindfulness Meditation, focusing on maintaining a level-headed presence in the present, reflecting upon Marcus Aurelius's quote: "Remember: Matter. How tiny your share of it. Time. How brief and fleeting your allotment of it."

Remember, there is no one-size-fits-all in Stoic Yoga. Continual improvement and adaptive change are integral. Listen to your body, respect its boundaries, permit yourself to limitlessly explore, and

customize your journey. In Stoicism and yoga, you are in the pursuit
of a union of mind and body that celebrates resilience, balance, and
tranquility. Unleash this power, and you will discover strength you
never knew existed.

Chapter 5. Unfolding the Path to Inner Strength

"Inner strength" is often perceived as an abstract and distant concept, hard to define and ever harder to attain. Yet, theoretically as well as practically, it forms the critical foundation of an enriching and fulfilling life. This chapter unfolds the path to the discovery, development, and nurturing of this elusive inner strength through the fusion of Stoic philosophy and Yoga practices, both deeply rooted in wisdom spanning across centuries.

5.1. Begin at the Mind's Crucible

Understanding inner strength begins at the very crucible of perceptions: our mind. The Stoics propound that our reactions and responses to life circumstances are directed by our minds, our perception of events, rather than the events themselves. Why is this important? Grappling with this core principle allows us to acknowledge that we have control over our minds and hence our reactions, setting the stage for resilience and internal resolve.

On the other hand, the practice of Yoga promotes the attainment of a balanced and disciplined mind. Seated meditation and asanas (Yogic postures) aim to observe, control, and eventually still the mind. Through this, we develop a profound sense of awareness of our body and mind, which in turn bolsters our mental fortitude.

A powerful alignment of the Stoic principle of mind control and the Yogic practice of mindful awareness can begin the journey to inner strength. This relationship can be further understood through a three-step path:

1. Acknowledge: Realize that events in life are neutral – they have no intrinsic value. They are layered with meaning based on our

perceptions.

2. Accept: Understand that our response to these events is within our control.

3. Act: Instead of getting swayed by the fluctuations of the mind, direct your focus on maintaining equanimity and worked through thought process.

5.2. Your Physical Dimension, Your Fortitude

The exterior strength of the body reflects your interior strength. Stoic philosophy suggests our external environment, including physical form, is transient. But it does not undermine the importance of caring for the physical form. Marcus Aurelius, a well-regarded Stoic philosopher, believed in treating the body with respect.

Yoga, too, lays emphasis on physical discipline through asanas. As we mindfully practice these postures, they offer more than just physical benefits – they equip us with the ability to face discomfort with grace, to moderate our reactions to physical stress, and to appreciate the impermanent nature of our physical being.

Combined, both Stoic and yogic practices enrich us with the revelation that physical discomfort or hardship does not equal suffering unless we so perceive it.

Here are some Yoga poses you can begin with:

1. Tadasana (Mountain pose): Teaches us to stand firm and grounded.

2. Virabhadrasana (Warrior pose): Develops courage and resilience.

3. Savasana (Corpse pose): Aids in physical relaxation and mental surrender.

Practicing these poses with stoic principles in mind can let you experience physical discomfort, understand its fleeting nature, and build a mind-body connection that imparts durability.

5.3. In The Still Waters of Inner Reflection

Inner strength is not only about resilience in face of adversity but also about taking the time to retreat into the self, for inner reflection. Stoic meditation or premeditatio malorum encourages reflecting on adversities that might occur in the future, allowing us to prepare for them, thereby cultivating resilience and tranquillity.

Similarly, Yoga meditation or Dhyana offers the practice of inward reflection. It cultivates the inner silence and tranquility required to access the deeper recesses of our being, where our true strength lies.

Calm, collected, concentrated – these states are achieved when we still the pond of our mind and allow the mud to settle. It's then that the clear waters of inner strength become noticeably clear. Engage in daily quiet reflection with these simple steps:

1. Choose a quiet, distraction-free space.

2. Meditate with a calm and open mind.

3. Try to visualize adversities and your calm response to them.

4. When thoughts get overwhelming, always return to your breath.

You can experience this powerful practice as a calming reassurance, a quiet validation of your capacity to live equanimously amid chaos.

5.4. Resilience is a Practice

Undeniably, both Stoicism and Yoga advocate the importance of practice in cultivating inner strength. They do not promise immediate transformation; they offer tenets and practices to foster ongoing growth. This might seem like an arduous journey, but remember, the journey itself is the reward.

Focusing on this continuous journey rather than the destination allows us to be immersed in the present, a concept vital in both Stoicism and Yoga. It also teaches us to respect our failures, viewing them as opportunities for growth rather than setbacks. Maintaining a journal of your experiences and thoughts can be useful in tracking and learning from your journey.

Incorporate the Stoic Yoga practices within your everyday life; let it not be a practice in isolation. Let the wisdom breathe through your life, through your actions, decisions, responses, and reflections. Strengthened with time, these interconnected web of practices begin to form the solid foundation of inner strength.

Take up this enriching path today and uncover the rewarding reservoir of your potential, harness the transformative power of inner strength, and discern how resilient and robust your life becomes in the face of life's trials and tribulations. With this knowledge in hand and a determined heart, you are prepared to unveil the Stoic Yogic within.

Chapter 6. The Art of Serenity: Stoicism in Action

To kick off our exploration, we draw attention to the heart of stoic philosophy - the principle of serenity. This principle hinges on understanding the world, accepting it as it is, and earnestly undertaking your role in it, immune to the turbulence of external influences. It's about partnering reason with nature's course, shunning fear, and embracing the journey of life from a fortitude of calm.

6.1. Serenity through Understanding

The stoics boldly declared that the path to serenity necessitates a profound understanding of life and our universe. A serene state of mind, to them, stemmed from the realization that certain elements in life, predominantly the ones outside of one's influence, should not be allowed to disturb one's tranquility.

This understanding draws from one of the core principles of Stoicism – the dichotomy of control. It focuses on categorizing life occurrences into two distinct bins – the ones we control and the ones we don't. Thus, the first step towards serenity, according to Stoicism, is acknowledging and accepting this dichotomy. Aligning our actions and reactions based on this understanding forms a fundamental part of our journey towards serenity.

Emblematically, the Stoic sage Epictetus postulated, "We should always be asking ourselves: 'Is this something that is, or is not, in my control?'". By steadily focusing our mental energy on elements within our capacity to change, we achieve a sense of peace, a harmonious serenity that springs from within.

6.2. The Doctrine of Acceptance

Embracing the concept of acceptance is elemental in applying stoicism in daily life. For the Stoics, acceptance was not a submissive resignation to fate, but a proactive affirmation of reality. It involves recognizing that change is a relentless constant and that adversity is an integral part of existence.

Epictetus again provides guidance, "Don't demand that things happen as you wish, but wish that they happen as they do happen, and you will go on well". In the face of trials, we don't merely endure but actively engage with them, seeing them as life's training grounds to build upon our inner strength and develop our wisdom.

It is here that acceptance converges with yogic philosophy, a practice deeply rooted in non-resistance, harmony, and acceptance of the present moment, whatever it might bring. Yoga teaches us to listen to our body, draw strength from it, and harmonise our spirit with the cosmic order - reinforcing the stoic objective of attaining serenity.

6.3. Cultivating Indifference to Indifferents

A key facet of Stoicism is developing an indifference to "indifferents,"- the Stoic concept of things outside our control. Wealth, reputation, health, and even life and death fall in this category. This does not advocate apathy, instead, it promotes a conscious detachment from the anxiety and stress these external factors often induce.

Marcus Aurelius, another noteworthy Stoic philosopher, and the Roman Emperor from AD 161 to 180, consistently instructed himself to remain unmoved by external occurrences, stating, "You have power over your mind – not outside events. Realize this, and you will find strength".

Embracing this idea of indifference challenges us to regulate our reactions to the undulating dynamics of the universe. It's about maintaining an equanimous state of mind, always.

6.4. Stoic Virtues for Serenity

Integral to Stoic philosophy are the cardinal virtues of Wisdom, Courage, Justice, and Temperance – building blocks to serenity in Stoic beliefs. By imbibing these virtues, we mold ourselves to become immune from the perturbations of life, standing as unwavering as an oak amidst a storm.

Stoic virtues coalesce beautifully with the yogic Yamas and Niyamas (observances and ethical guidelines); non-violence echoes courage, truthfulness embodies wisdom, contentment resonates with temperance, and purity reflects justice. Combining these systems, we realize an enriching symbiosis that augments mental and spiritual growth, fostering a lasting serenity.

6.5. Tools for Building Serenity

Stoicism provides practical tools, such as negative visualization and voluntary discomfort, to construct a strong foundation for serenity. Negative visualization trains our mind to anticipate adverse conditions, making us better prepared and less affected when they occur.

Voluntary discomfort is deliberately exposing ourselves to uncomfortable situations to toughen our mental resilience. Pair these exercises with Yoga's breathing techniques (Pranayama) and physical postures (Asanas), and we boost our endurance levels, priming ourselves to stay serene under any circumstance.

6.6. Conclusion: Bridging Stoicism with Daily Life

To embrace the art of serenity, we need to internalize the stoic wisdom of understanding, acceptance, and indifference. Nurturing stoic virtues and employing stoic tools in our response to life's vicissitudes help fortify this state of serenity.

As we blend stoicism with the daily practice of yoga, a symbiotic harmony is formed, amplifying our journey towards mental peace and inner strength. It is this harmonious blend that can guide us throughout life, enabling us to live in sync with nature while we navigate the world as tranquil souls, undisturbed by external chaos.

The journey to serenity is full of introspection, courage, wisdom, and a willingness to accept. But, as we steadily walk this path, embracing its lessons, we will surely find ourselves rooted in an unshakeable tranquility, an unwavering fortress of serenity.

Chapter 7. Inciting Physical Wellness with Yoga

The exploration of yoga begins with an understanding of its origin and philosophy. Yoga, an ancient practice approximately five thousand years old, hails from India. Initially, its focus was not physical fitness as in modern times, but rather a path to spiritual enlightenment. Over the centuries, yoga has blossomed into a multifaceted discipline, with physical wellness being a prominent aspect of the practice.

7.1. The Basics of Physical Yoga

At a superficial glance, yoga might seem merely an array of bodily poses known as asana. However, asana, one of the eight limbs of yoga, is far more profound than simple body contortions. It is a doorway to meld mind, body, and spirit, instilling a deep-seated sense of unity and wholeness that allows us to resonate with our highest potential.

Incorporating yoga into your daily regimen is a decision that pays dividends in terms of physical health. With regular practice, you begin to experience increased flexibility, enhanced muscle strength and tone, improved respiration, and a substantial boost in energy levels. This is a result of not just the physical poses but also the controlled, conscious breathing that underlies every yoga practice.

7.2. Unraveling Asana: A Closer Look

Asanas, the physical poses of yoga, serve as the bedrock of the practice. There are hundreds of asanas, each designed to target different parts of the body. Although they vary in complexity and effort required, they all share a common denominator: the union of the body and mind through controlled movement.

Here's a basic asciidoc table of some common yoga asanas.

Name of Asana	Physical Benefits
Tadasana (Mountain Pose)	Enhances posture, strengthens thighs, knees, and ankles
Vrikshasana (Tree Pose)	Stabilizes and improves balance, strengthens legs
Adho Mukha Svanasana (Downward Dog)	Strengthens arms, legs, stretches the spine
Bhujangasana (Cobra Pose)	Improves flexibility, tones the abdomen
Savasana (Corpse Pose)	Promotes relaxation and calms the mind

7.3. Yoga Beyond Asana

While asana is a fundamental aspect of yoga, other components, such as pranayama (breathing exercises) and meditation, complement it and maximize its efficacy. Pranayama and meditation foster a calm and focused mind, vital for overall physical wellness.

Pranayama involves various breathing techniques designed to control the flow of prana, our vital life force. Calming pranayamas such as Sheetali and Anulom Vilom can lower stress levels, ensuring better physical health. On the other hand, energy-boosting pranayamas like Kapalbhati and Bhastrika can stimulate the metabolic rate and aid in weight loss.

Meditation concludes most yoga sessions, serving as a time of stillness and reflection that allows the benefits of the asana practice to permeate our body. It creates a space to tune into our thought patterns and emotions, promoting mental wellness which translates into better physical health.

7.4. Integrating Yoga into Your Daily Routine

Bringing yoga into your everyday life doesn't have to be a daunting task. Start small, with just a few minutes a day, gradually extending the duration as per your comfort level. Whether you're a morning bird who can fit in a session at dawn or a night owl who prefers to stretch out the day's stress after work, choose a time that works for your routine.

Seek the guidance of a qualified yoga instructor initially to ensure that you are performing the asanas correctly. Once you're comfortable, you can continue practicing independently, using resources such as online lessons or yoga books.

Remember, consistency is arguably more crucial than the length of your practice. Even a short daily session is better than a lengthy session once a fortnight. Slow and steady progress is the essence of the yoga journey.

7.5. Navigating Potential Challenges

Just as with any new endeavor, you might face challenges when commencing your yoga journey — physical discomfort with certain postures, difficulty in quieting the mind during meditation, or even a lack of time. Remember, yoga is not about perfection; it's about progress. Listening to your body's cues and progressing at your own pace might be challenging initially but will contribute to a more sustainable and beneficial practice in the long run.

Yoga is fundamentally a journey inward, a pathway leading you to better understand, nurture, and celebrate your body. When followed consistently and mindfully, the path laid by yoga can open the doors to a realm of physical wellbeing beyond mere fitness, a state of holistic health imbued with robust vitality and remarkable resilience. As you embark on this journey, remember to be patient with yourself and savor every breath and movement.

Chapter 8. Stoic Yoga: A Bridge Between Mind and Body

The exploration of the synergy between Stoicism and Yoga begins with an understanding of the two foundational pillars.

8.1. The Pillars of Stoic Yoga

Stoicism and Yoga, two ancient philosophies and practices, hail from distant corners of the world - Greece and India respectively - yet they share a striking similarity, the pursuit of liberation through wisdom, virtue, and self-discipline. One might even consider Stoicism as the Yoga of the West and vice versa.

---- Stoicism This Hellenistic philosophy taught that virtue (the highest good) is based on knowledge. The wise live in harmony with the divine Nature, treating whatever life presents them with equanimity. Stoicism emphasizes four cardinal virtues which are: wisdom, courage, justice, and temperance (moderation).

---- Yoga In Sanskrit, Yoga means 'union,' often interpreted as the union of mind, body, and spirit. It consists of eight stages or limbs culminating in Samadhi - the state of intense concentration and blissful awareness. Each stage, in order, teaches how to control one's body, mind, and ultimately, merge with the divine.

Stoic Yoga then is not inherently a novel concept; it's a unification of two systems that fundamentally aim towards the same goal: inner peace, tranquility and an understanding of one's place in the natural order of life.

8.2. Practicing Stoic Yoga: The Bridge To Mind-Body Connection

Stoic Yoga introduces an empowering blend of Physical Asana (Yoga Postures) and Stoic Philosophical Meditations and Reflections. This amalgamation deftly serves to bridge the gap between the harmony of body and mind.

---- Asana and Stoic Virtue The training of the physical body is as much a virtue as the training of one's mind, for it reflects the respect we accord to the vessel housing our spirituality. Emphasizing tranquility, the physical training in Stoic Yoga involves practicing mindful postures inspired from Yoga. Each Asana aims to reinforce the four stoic virtues: wisdom, courage, justice, and temperance, hence fostering resilience amidst adversities.

For example, the Mountain Pose (Tadasana), a foundational standing posture in yoga, can be correlated to the virtue of wisdom. This pose encourages one to stand tall, steady, immovable like a mountain - displaying stability, clarity, and groundedness - qualities synonymous with wisdom.

---- Mental Equilibrium: Meditating and Reflecting Here, Stoic philosophy comes into play, utilising its notions of self-reflection and meditation to strengthen the mind. Stoic meditation differs from other meditation forms. It asks practitioners to reflect on events, their responses to them, and how they could be handled better. It's more an exercise of the mind to achieve mental resilience than a process to empty or silence the mind.

It's also important to note that Stoic Yoga places great emphasis on journaling as a form of meditation. It encourages practitioners to write down their reflections, observations and thoughts as they traverse through their journey. This aids in maintaining a clear account of personal growth and the wisdom gathered.

8.3. Channeling Stoic Yoga For Inner Transformation

Practicing Stoic Yoga leads the seeker through a profound internal metamorphosis, a transformation into the best possible version of oneself.

---- Tranquility amidst Chaos The unique amalgamation of Stoic philosophy and yogic practices enables us to remain tranquil amidst turbulence. The external world's chaos ceases to be the trigger for our reactions; instead, our inner compass guides us. Our emotional resilience nourishes us, allowing us to maintain our calmness in every situation.

---- Conscious Decisions With the practice of Stoic Yoga, our decisions cease to be impulsive; instead, they become conscious choices. We feel and understand the gentle whisperings of our intuition and respond, instead of react, to situations.

To exemplify, Asanas encourage mindfulness—the acute awareness of our body and breath makes us conscious of the moment, while Stoic reflections allow us a deeper assimilation of our past actions and future decisions.

8.4. Conclusion: Stoic Yoga - A Journey Towards Equilibrium

Stoic Yoga is more than just a physical or philosophical exercise; it's a way of life—a path towards inner strength, tranquility, and resilience. It's the bridge that harmonizes the wisdom from the West with the holistic approach from the East to help individuals lead a balanced life amidst the chaos of the world.

In conclusion, the union of Stoicism and Yoga gifts us the knowledge and power to control what's within us: our actions, reactions, and attitudes, thus guiding us to live life to its fullest potential. So endeavor onto this loving merge of philosophies and practices, and unleash the profound depths of self-understanding and harmony.

Chapter 9. Exercise Routines: Aligning Stoic Thought with Yoga Asanas

Incorporating Stoic principles into your yoga practice is not just about physical postures; it's adopting a rich philosophical mindset that focuses on virtues, mindfulness, and conscious living. This alignment offers an incredible opportunity to develop a more balanced inner life and expand your capacity for resilience and equanimity.

9.1. Understanding Stoicism in Yoga

Stoicism, an ancient Greek philosophy, teaches us to focus on what's within our control and let go of what's not. For Stoics, happiness doesn't derive from external circumstances but how we choose to perceive them. In the realm of yoga, this principle can be directly applied; your asanas are not measured by how they look externally but by your internal experience during the practice.

The Stoics defined four cardinal virtues: wisdom, courage, justice, and temperance. These virtues can become a corner piece of your yoga practice. By interpreting them through yoga, you create a practice that nurtures your inner self.

9.2. Wisdom: Discerning the Essential

Wisdom in Stoicism is about understanding and focusing on what is within our control. It encourages us to let go of our obsession with perfection and external validation while guiding us on the path of purposeful acceptance.

In your yoga practice, apply wisdom by concentrating on your experience rather than the outcome. For instance, when practicing Tadasana (Mountain Pose), your focus shouldn't be on achieving the 'perfect pose'. Instead, pay attention to your alignment, your breath, and the strength in your core. This is what is within your control, not the external image you create.

9.3. Courage: Strength Beyond Asanas

Courage in Stoicism does not merely relate to physical bravery, but also to a mental state. It matters how you respond when faced with discomfort or difficulty, showing resilience in the face of challenging poses or holding asanas for longer.

In Pigeon Pose (Eka Pada Rajakapotasana), you might experience discomfort. Rather than escaping from this discomfort, exercise courage by consciously breathing into these tense areas and slowly releasing the tension.

9.4. Justice: Balance and Fairness to Self

Justice in Stoicism refers to our relationships with others, and importantly, with ourselves. It's about acting with integrity and honesty.

In yoga, justice can be reflected in your self regard. Recognize the need for self-care, rest, and balance. You can adjust your practice to meet your needs, balancing active asanas with restorative ones. Practice Child's Pose (Balasana) to rest and rejuvenate your mind and body.

9.5. Temperance: Moderation in All Things

Temperance, for Stoics, is the practice of moderation and self-restraint. It's a delicate dance between effort and ease.

In yoga, temperance is mirrored in the concept of "Ahimsa" or non-harming. Pushing your body excessively to achieve certain postures can lead to harm. Allow temperance to guide you. During the Dolphin Pose (Ardha Pincha Mayurasana), if your shoulders start to ache, it's an indicator to exercise restraint and ease out of the pose.

9.6. Stoic-Yoga Blend for a Week

Now, blending these philosophical insights with your yoga practice, here is a week-long yoga routine that encapsulates these Stoic principles into daily yoga practice.

1. Monday: Warm up with Sun Salutations (Surya Namaskar). Go with the flow of your body and cultivate mindfulness regarding what you feel in each pose. Progress to Warrior II (Virabhadrasana II) to exercise courage.

2. Tuesday: Begin with Tree pose (Vrksasana) to foster a sense of balance. Transition into Triangle Pose (Trikonasana) for depth and introspection.

3. Wednesday: Open your session with a gentle Camel pose (Ustrasana). Develop your practice further with Crow Pose (Bakasana), helping to build physical and mental fortitude.

4. Thursday: Start with Bridge pose (Setu Bandha Sarvangasana) for internal reflection. Move towards Extended Side Angle Pose (Utthita Parsvakonasana), playing with the balance of energy.

5. Friday: Commence with Cat-Cow pose (Marjaryasana-Bitilasana) to build mindfulness. Advance to Seated Forward Bend

(Paschimottanasana) for quiet introspection.

6. Saturday: Open with Gentle Supine Twist (Supta Matsyendrasana) to kindle the sense of justice to the body. Move on to Cobra Pose (Bhujangasana) for heartfelt awareness of self.

7. Sunday: A day for integration and temperance. Begin with Corpse Pose (Savasana), facilitating an absorbing meditation. Transition into Lotus Pose (Padmasana), centering your focus inward and embodying tranquility.

In essence, Stoic Yoga isn't just a physical exercise; it's a lifestyle, a state of mind. It's working within your limits, embracing difficulties, and moving towards a state of resilient calm. Adopt this Stoic-Yoga blend into your daily routines, and reimagine the way you approach yoga and life itself. Remember, Excellence, as per Stoic philosophy, is not a single act but a habit, the holistic practice of bringing wisdom, courage, justice, and temperance into your yoga and beyond.

Chapter 10. Navigating Life's Challenges: Stoic Yoga in Everyday Life

Embracing the central tenets of Stoic philosophy in conjunction with Yoga is akin to embarking on a journey that enables one to effectively navigate the prevalent storms of life by fostering resilience and promoting mental balance. This chapter aims to shed light on the profound synergies between these two disciplines, determining precisely how we can leverage their combined power to effectively overcome life's challenges.

10.1. Stoic Philosophy: An Overview

Stoic philosophy hinges on the belief that tranquility of mind and soul can be achieved, irrespective of the external circumstances. Our inner state, according to the Stoics, depends primarily on our attitudes, judgments, and responses, rather than the events themselves. The philosophy encourages us to focus our energies on aspects we can influence while accepting those beyond our control.

===Unfolding Yoga Tradition

Yoga, with its rich tradition spanning thousands of years, similary aims at unifying mind, body, and spirit. It empowers individuals to attain a state of balance and harmony by cultivating mindfulness, building physical strength and flexibility, and fostering inner peace. Yoga cultivates a centered and grounded state of being, allowing yogis to maintain calm and composure when confronted by life's trials.

===Harnessing the Power of Stoic Yoga

Combining the wisdom of Stoicism with the physical and mental discipline of Yoga, you foster a potent synergy that imbues resilience and tranquility. Practicing Stoic Yoga in everyday life involves mastering the ability to maintain composure and reasoning ability amid adversity.

10.2. Cultivating Mind-body Cohesion

The first step in integrating Stoic philosophy and Yoga is to foster a connection between the body and mind. Physical practices like asanas, pranayama, and meditation promote this balance, initiating a state of mindfulness where the mind attunes to the body and vice versa.

For instance, while holding a challenging pose, focus not on the discomfort but consider it a reminder of the transient nature of all things (a Stoic principle). Elucidating how you perceive and react to physical distress can significantly influence your responses to emotional or psychological upheaval in everyday life.

10.3. Practicing Acceptance

Life inevitably presents us various trials. Acceptance - the ability to accept things as they are, especially those beyond our control - is central to both Stoicism and Yoga. Building acceptance involves altering the way we perceive and respond to adversity.

For instance, rather than resisting or struggling against a demanding Yoga pose, one could instead accept the discomfort, observe it without judgment, and stay present. By paralleling this practice with life's challenges, one can learn to handle adversity with grace and equanimity.

10.4. Achieving Mental Equilibrium

Practicing stoic yoga invites us to explore and reframe our thoughts and attitudes, leading to a tranquil mind. Mindfulness meditation and self-reflective practices akin to Stoic 'journaling' can aid in achieving this mental equilibrium.

While meditating, observe your thoughts and emotions from a detached perspective, keeping the stoic idea of "some things are in our control and others not" at the forefront. This will help train the mind to stay uneffected by the impressions and impulses that would ordinarily elicit a reactionary response.

10.5. Building Resilience

Yoga poses that test your strength and balance metaphorically represent the challenges life throws at us. Regular practice renders flexibility and resilience, not just physically, but also mentally. When coupled with Stoic principles of responding to hardship rationally and calmly, it strengthens the capacity to resist or recover from difficulties.

10.6. Conclusion

Indeed, applying Stoic Yoga principles to everyday life does not merely offer one a breather amidst life's storm but quite literally augments one's ability to navigate life's turbulences. It is about building a fortress within, one that is not easily disrupted by external events. Stoic Yoga thus provides a structured, practical approach towards achieving a harmonious, resilient, and serene existence.

Chapter 11. An Ongoing Journey: Next Steps in the Practice of Stoic Yoga

Stoic Yoga, as a practice, isn't a mere destination—it's an ongoing journey. You constantly embrace new perspectives, push your limits, and evolve on your path towards extraordinary resilience and tranquility. As you delve into the venture of Stoic Yoga, it's crucial that you plan your future steps. This is mainly about cultivating your Stoic Yoga routine, knowing how Stoic philosophy can integrate with the different yoga asanas (postures), and nurturing a mindset of tranquility amid chaos.

11.1. Deepening Your Stoic Yoga Routine

To strengthen your Stoic Yoga practice, establish routines that enable you to internalize and live the principles of both realms. Expanding your practice requires continuous bouts of introspection, physiological discipline, and mental conditioning.

An effective Stoic Yoga routine embodies three core elements - yoga asanas, breathing exercises, and Stoic reflections. Start with a gentle warm-up before progressing into a series of yoga postures, steadily synchronizing your breath with each movement. Cap off your session with a short period of Stoic meditation that allows you to reflect on the practice and draw key insights from it.

Remember, the key to a successful routine is consistency – make it non-negotiable. Establish a set time in your daily schedule and make sure to practice at least for a brief period, no matter what. It's not about the length of the practice, but the continuity that breeds profound transformations.

11.2. Integrating Stoic Philosophy into Yoga Asanas

Integral to the practice of Stoic Yoga is the amalgamation of Stoic philosophy and yoga postures. Each asana, when combined with the tenets of Stoicism, can invite a greater sense of tranquility and fortitude within you.

Stoic philosophers believed in the power of rational thought over passions, and this philosophy can serve as a mental guide during your yoga flow. For instance, while holding a difficult pose such as 'Warrior 2', remind yourself of the Stoic ingrained virtue of courage - facing adversity without succumbing to discomfort.

11.3. Cultivating a Stoic Mindset Amid Chaos

The Stoic Yoga journey isn't limited to your yoga mat—it extends into every aspect of your life. The ultimate goal is to cultivate a stoic mindset—maintaining tranquility amid chaos, embracing the impermanence of life, and understanding what's within your control.

To cultivate the stoic mindset, start small. Begin by observing your reactions to everyday inconveniences - being stuck in traffic, experiencing a sudden shift in weather, or encountering a mental block at work. Whenever you catch yourself feeling agitated, frustrated, or restless, take a moment to pause and remind yourself of the Stoic principle of accepting things outside our control.

11.4. Measuring Your Progress

The transformative journey of Stoic Yoga isn't linear, and measuring progress can be a complex task. Some days, you might feel immensely tranquil, and on others, you might struggle with maintaining emotional equilibrium, especially in chaotic situations.

Instead of letting this discourage you, use it as a tool for self-reflections. Record your experiences in a Stoic journal – what were your highs, what were the lows, and how did you respond? Analyze these entries over time and notice patterns, improvements, and areas that need attention. Regularly writing in a journal also fortifies your engagement with the Stoic Yoga practice, making it an indispensable part of your life.

11.5. The Path of Continued Learning

The Stoic Yogi is a perpetual student who continually seeks knowledge and insight. Immersing yourself in further learning can propel your journey forward. Read books, listen to podcasts, or attend workshops about Stoicism and Yoga. Plato once said, "Ignorance, the root and the stem of every evil." Ignorance can't be an ally on your path to inner strength and tranquility.

The Stoic Yoga journey is a wonderful blend of physical resilience and mental fortitude. It's a lifelong voyage of self-discovery, wisdom, and resilience. As you tread on this path, nourish your practice with patience, persistence, consistency, curiosity, and acceptance. Devote yourself to the grueling yet fulfilling training of mind and body. This wouldn't just fortify your resolve to deal with life's vicissitudes; it will also foster an invincible spirit that no circumstance can tarnish.